Thyroid Diet

How to Improve Thyroid Disorders, Manage Thyroid Symptoms, Lose Weight, and Improve Your Metabolism through Diet!

Table Of Contents

Introduction 1

Chapter 1: The Thyroid and its Common Disorders 2

Chapter 2: Importance of Iodine.. 7

Chapter 3: Foods to Avoid.. 12

Chapter 4: Other Nutrients for Thyroid Health..................... 14

Chapter 5: Tips on Planning a Thyroid-Friendly Diet 21

Conclusion 25

Introduction

I want to thank you and congratulate you for downloading the book, "Thyroid Diet: How to Improve Thyroid Disorders, Manage Thyroid Symptoms, Lose Weight, and Improve Your Metabolism through Diet!".

This book contains helpful information about thyroid disorders, and how they can be improved through dietary changes!

You will soon learn about the different thyroid disorders that people suffer from, their causes, and also how to improve and prevent them.

Thyroid disorders are primarily the result of dietary insufficiencies, and as such this book will be focusing on diet. You will soon discover the different foods that cause thyroid disorders, along with those that help to prevent and cure them.

This book will explain to you tips and techniques that will allow you to begin successfully managing and recovering from your thyroid disorder with the help of food! By making the simple dietary changes suggested within this guide, you'll be able to improve your thyroid disorder, or potentially prevent yourself from developing one in the first place!

Thanks again for downloading this book, I hope you enjoy it!

Chapter 1:
The Thyroid and its Common Disorders

The thyroid is one of the body's endocrine glands. It is found in the neck area, below the Adam's apple and just in front of the trachea. It has a butterfly-like shape with the left and right lobes linked together by a narrow gland tissue in the middle called an isthmus.

The thyroid produces a number of thyroid hormones that influence the body's metabolism, protein generation, internal temperature, and holistic development. The two main thyroid hormones produced are triiodothyronine (T_3) and thyroxine (T_4), which is also sometimes called tetraiodothyronine. Sufficient thyroid hormone generation is vital for brain development, especially of infants and children. It is also essential for prenatal development as adequate maternal thyroid hormones (hormones coming from the mother) are needed to protect the fetus from any neurodevelopmental disorders.

With all of these important functions, it is clear that the thyroid is one of the most essential organs of the human body. And like all the other organs, the thyroid is not immune from illnesses and disorders that specifically affect it.

The most common types of thyroid disorders are the following:

1. Goiter – is the conventional term used for the enlargement of the thyroid gland. There are many causes of thyroid swelling, but statistics show that more than 90 percent of goiters around the world are caused by iodine deficiency. Other possible causes of goiter are congenital hypothyroidism, repeated intake of goitrogens (foods that suppress the absorption of iodine by the body), Basedow syndrome (more popularly known as Graves' disease), Hashimoto's thyroiditis, pituitary gland disease, and adverse reactions to drugs or other medications.

Not all cases of goiter may show any symptoms, although the typical ones are a noticeable bulging of the neck, having a hard time breathing or swallowing, a firm feeling around the throat, coughing, and sometimes huskiness of voice.

Treatment for goiters varies depending on the root cause. Some benign goiters that have only mild swelling are usually not treated at all and are allowed to heal on their own. With the addition of more iodine in the standard, everyday diet, particularly with the increased availability of iodized salt, the incidence of goiter worldwide has significantly gone down over the years.

2. Hyperthyroidism – is a disorder in which the thyroid gland excessively produces thyroid hormones that are no longer needed by the body. This overproduction is a problem, because when there is an abundance of T_3 and T_4 hormones in the body, its metabolism is drastically stimulated. This makes a person lose weight rapidly, sometimes dangerously, and causes them to experience abnormal sweating, irregular heartbeat, and anxiety attacks.

The common causes of hyperthyroidism are iodine oversufficiency, swelling of the thyroid gland that leaks out excess thyroid hormones, tumors in the testes (for men) or ovary (for women), and the over consumption of tetraiodothyronine (T_4 hormones) found in dietary supplements or medicines that are prescribed to treat hypothyroidism.

This condition is somewhat difficult to diagnose as most of its major symptoms are also common to other diseases, such as abrupt weight loss, rapid heartbeat (typically over a hundred beats per minute), heart palpitations, frequent mood swings, anxiousness, shaking of the hands and fingers, increased sweating, insomnia, tiredness and weariness, and thinning of the hair and skin. Most of the time, though, there are no symptoms at all, which is another reason why it is hard to detect this kind of thyroid disorder.

Fortunately, there are dietary treatments to improve the symptoms of hyperthyroidism. Consuming the right amounts of calories, sodium, vitamins, minerals, and other nutrients could help prevent the production of too much thyroid hormones in the body.

3. Hypothyroidism – is the exact opposite of hyperthyroidism as it is the condition when the thyroid gland does not produce enough thyroid hormones for the body to utilize. Again, this other extreme is a problem because without enough T_3 and T_4 hormones in the system, the body's metabolism becomes too slow. It results in weight gain, fatigue, physical and mental weaknesses, and sometimes depression.

For little children, insufficient thyroid hormones critically affect physical growth and intellectual development, which could sometimes lead to cretinism. Prolonged and untreated hypothyroidism could also cause other kinds of conditions and illnesses such as peripheral neuropathy, heart disease, myxedema, infertility, and some mental disorders.

This inadequate production of thyroid hormones is typically caused by treatments and medications for hyperthyroidism, treatments and medications for heart diseases and mental disorders, the complete or partial removal of the thyroid gland via surgery to remove cancer, and having insufficient iodine in the diet.

Similar to other thyroid disorders, one of the most effective ways of alleviating the symptoms of hypothyroidism is by having proper food and nutritional intake as well.

4. Thyroid Cancer – This is one of the rarest forms of cancers and is normally treatable. It is easily curable because its onset is easy to detect. There are also many effective remedies available today. However, it can still recur even after a lot of years of successful treatment.

Medical experts and practitioners still cannot pinpoint the exact causes of thyroid cancer. However, it is widely speculated to be the result of DNA changes brought about by old age. It could also be genetic or hereditary in nature. It is also observed that people who have been subjected to a lot of past radiation therapies in the chest, neck, and head, have a higher risk of obtaining thyroid cancer later on in their lives.

The common symptoms are a noticeable bump in the neck, soreness of the neck and the inner ears, difficulty in breathing and swallowing, huskiness of voice, and recurrent coughing that is unrelated to ordinary flu, cold, or any lung disease.

The conventional treatments for thyroid cancer are surgery and radiation therapy, although having the right diet could also help in relieving its symptoms.

5. Thyroiditis – is a term used to refer to a wide array of conditions that cause the inflammation of the thyroid gland. The common causes of inflammation are either an autoimmune disorder or a viral disease that specifically attacks the thyroid.

Similar to hyperthyroidism, thyroiditis' symptoms are also the signs and symptoms of other common diseases. This is why it takes a few more tests before it can be diagnosed correctly. Some of these indications are tiredness, weight gain, nausea, depression, drying of the skin, and infrequent bowel movement. In extreme cases, the inflammation of the thyroid causes the body temperature to drop, the areas around the eyes to become puffy, and the heart rate to become very slow which may continue to the point of failing.

Treatments are given to a patient according to what kind of thyroiditis they're suffering from. Among the treatment options are surgery, and the taking of antibiotics or other medications. Consuming the right amounts of the recommended foods could also help a lot in preventing the acquisition of this disease.

Managing Thyroid Disorders using Proper Diet

Your food intake can affect the health and function of your thyroid more than you may know. That is why it is necessary to watch what you eat in order to keep your thyroid gland in peak condition.

The next chapters will talk more about the foods to eat, foods to avoid, and how to plan the right diet to help treat and prevent each of the common thyroid disorders mentioned above.

Chapter 2:
Importance of Iodine

An insufficiency of iodine in the diet is the number one cause of basically all types of thyroid disorders. This is especially true in poor nations where a significant shortage in food supply is always experienced. Thus, its citizens are not conscious of, or are not interested in, consuming a proper diet. However, in countries where there is more awareness, and iodized salt is cheap and readily available in the market, cases of thyroid disorders are actually very low.

Importance of Iodine

Iodine in the blood is taken by the thyroid gland in order to activate the process of producing thyroid hormones. When there is not enough iodine in the bloodstream, another endocrine gland called the pituitary gland (found in the brain) communicates to the rest of the body that there is a said insufficiency. When this happens, the pituitary gland releases a hormone called Thyroid-Stimulating Hormone, or TSH, which forces the thyroid gland to produce more T_3 and T_4 hormones. This is harmful because it causes the thyroid gland to become enlarged or swollen, which then causes different kinds of thyroid problems.

Therefore, it is highly important to have sufficient iodine in the body for the general health and strength of the thyroid gland. The recommended daily intake of iodine is 150 micrograms.

To give you an idea of the proper amount and the right kinds of food to eat to prevent iodine deficiency, below is a list of iodine-rich foods.

List of Iodine-rich Foods

Aside from regularly using iodized salt in preparing your meals, here are some foods that you may incorporate in your daily diet in order for you to increase your iodine intake:

1. Milk – although this beverage is more popular for providing your body with the essential nutrients of vitamin D and calcium, it is actually a significant source of iodine as well. A glass of milk includes 56 micrograms of iodine, which is around 37 percent of the total recommended daily intake. Other dairy products such as organic cheese and yogurt are also high in iodine.

2. Yogurt – a cup of plain yogurt has about 150 micrograms of iodine, which is 100 percent of the recommended daily consumption. Having yogurt every morning for breakfast is a good idea as it also provides a healthy dose of protein and calcium.

3. Cheddar cheese – an ounce of this type of cheese provides approximately 12 micrograms of iodine. The portion should be quite small, as the ounce serving contains 452 calories. Still, it is still a nice option to consider for cheese lovers.

4. Potatoes – this root crop is another abundant source of iodine. A regular medium-sized potato contains a whopping 60 micrograms of iodine. Preparing it baked or boiled is better than mashing it, as most of the dietary benefits of potatoes, such as potassium, vitamins, and fiber, are held in their skin. It is also better to only consume the organic kind, since the skin

of potatoes keep much of the pesticides used during its farming.

5. Hard-boiled egg – a large-sized hard-boiled egg can provide around 12 micrograms of iodine, or a little less than 10 percent of the recommended daily intake. Aside from that, eggs are also good antioxidants. They provide fair amounts of calcium, zinc, and vitamins D and A.

6. White pea bean – beans are generally good sources of iodine, but white pea beans have been found to be the most iodine-rich. A half cup of these beans will give you around 32 micrograms of iodine. Apart from that, they also contains high amounts of fiber that aids proper digestion. Also, unlike other canned products that normally lose their dietary values because of processing, canned white pea beans retain most of their nutrients even when processed or canned.

7. Cranberries – aside from being an effective antioxidant, cranberries are also a rich source of iodine. A single ounce of fresh cranberries has about 100 micrograms of iodine, which is almost the amount required for the recommended daily consumption. Cranberries provide moderate amounts of fiber, vitamin C, and manganese, and are also a rich source of phytochemicals that boost the cardiovascular and immune systems. Cranberry juice is also famous for being effective in preventing urinary tract infections. They are actually considered by most dieticians as one of the world's healthiest foods.

8. Strawberries – another fruit that contains a fairly good amount of iodine is the strawberry. One cup of fresh strawberries can give you about 15 micrograms of

iodine, exactly 10 percent of the recommended daily intake. Like cranberries, they are also a rich source of vitamin C, manganese, and phytochemicals.

9. Shrimp – as with all the other seafood, shrimps are a good source of iodine as well. A three-ounce portion contains 35 micrograms of iodine, or 23 percent of the recommended daily consumption. It can also provide sufficient amounts of calcium, protein, and omega 3 fatty acids. Shrimps are also deemed beneficial to the circulatory system as they enhance the proportion of LDL and HDL cholesterol levels and significantly reduce triglycerides.

10. Lobster – lobsters are also great sources of iodine as a 100-gram portion of it has 100 micrograms of iodine, or 67 percent of the recommended daily intake. They are also rich in iron, zinc, phosphorus, potassium, magnesium, calcium, and vitamins A, B2, B3, B6, and B12.

11. Tuna – this saltwater fish is rich in iodine and is an important source of omega 3 fatty acids as well. It contains 34 micrograms of iodine for every six ounce serving. When it comes to canned tuna, those that are prepared in oil have more iodine than those prepared in water. The other nutrients sufficiently provided by tuna are iron, protein, and vitamin D.

12. Cod – another saltwater fish that contains huge amounts of iodine is cod. Just a three-ounce portion has an incredible 99 micrograms of iodine, or about 66 percent of the recommended daily intake. Aside from that, cod liver oil also provides sufficient amounts of omega 3 fatty acids and vitamins A, D, and E.

13. Kelp – is a large seaweed found in the shallow parts of the ocean. Its iodine content is enormous. Just a mere quarter of an ounce contains 4,500 micrograms of iodine, which is 3,000 percent of the recommended daily intake. It is advised to eat only small servings at a time as it may result in an oversufficiency of iodine. Other species of kelp that have high concentrations of iodine are wakame (80 micrograms per tablespoon), arame (730 micrograms per tablespoon), hiziki (780 micrograms per tablespoon), and kombu (1,450 micrograms in every 1-inch portion).

14. Turkey meat – apart from having the most protein content for every ounce among all meats, it is also a good source of iodine. Three ounces contains 34 micrograms of iodine. It also gives a healthy dose of potassium, phosphorus, and B vitamins.

These are only some of the foods that are rich in iodine, and there are many more. It is also important to keep in mind, however, that the overconsumption of iodine is also not good for your thyroid health, which is why a balanced diet is needed.

Chapter 3:
Foods to Avoid

If there are food items that can improve the function of the thyroid gland, there are also certain food types that specifically contribute to its dysfunction. These food types should thus be avoided as much as possible. Some of these foods impede the thyroid's ability to get iodine from the blood, while others prevent the production of thyroid hormones itself. Either way, both are not useful to help keep the thyroid healthy and functioning properly. Below are some of the food products to avoid if you have a thyroid disorder.

1. Cruciferous vegetables such as cauliflower, broccoli, kale, Brussel sprouts, turnip, and cabbage. It is said that these veggies inhibit the absorption of iodine by the thyroid gland. It is not advised, however, to totally eliminate them from your diet as they do provide a lot of health benefits as well. To remove their anti-iodine effect on the body, simply shred or boil them before eating.

2. Any soy products such as soy beans, soy sauce, soy milk, and tofu. A study issued by the National Institutes of Health said that soy products have anti-thyroid characteristics that are intensified when a person is already suffering from an iodine deficiency. However, as long as you are eating enough iodine-rich foods, you can still consume these products for their specific dietary benefits, but in small amounts only.

3. Processed foods such as white sugar, white flour, and white bread.

4. Artificial sweeteners such as aspartame. Medical experts say that the regular consumption of aspartame leads to autoimmune diseases that affect the thyroid.

5. Gluten contained in wheat, barley, and rye, as well as in all processed foods. It is reported that it also causes autoimmune conditions that induce thyroid swelling.

6. Any fried or greasy food. Meats that are fatty, such as pork and beef, should also be avoided. Opt for friendlier sources of protein instead, like lentils, beans, milk, eggs, fish and other seafood.

7. Coffee, tea, soda, and other caffeinated products. You can consume them daily but only in small amounts.

8. Alcoholic drinks of any kind.

Since thyroid problems are most often caused by iodine deficiency, its prevention (as well as treatment if you already have it) begins by making sure that you have enough iodine in your daily food intake. This should be done in tandem with staying away from foods that lower its effectiveness.

Chapter 4:
Other Nutrients for Thyroid Health

As you may have already presumed, iodine is definitely not the only nutrient that can help to improve thyroid disorders. Although it is the main nutrient that the body needs to maintain good thyroid health, there are also other nutrients that support the thyroid gland and allow it to function well. Below are some of these nutrients and the most common food products that contain them.

1. **Selenium** – apart from iodine, selenium is considered as the most essential element for thyroid health. It helps the thyroid gland by regulating the production of thyroid hormones and the reusing of the body's excess iodine. It also benefits all of the body cells that specifically utilize thyroid hormones by converting thyroxine (T4) into the more active triiodothyronine (T3) for better metabolism function. Selenium also relieves social, chemical, and oxidative stress experienced by the thyroid.

    Without enough selenium in the body, the thyroid works in a constant state of stress, which could eventually break it down, making it detrimental to a person's overall wellbeing. Hypothyroidism is one of the major effects of insufficient selenium. Other effects include tiredness, depression, intellectual disability, cretinism for infants, and frequent miscarriages for women. Other diseases that come from selenium deficiency are Kashin-Beck disease and Keshan disease.

    Common selenium-rich foods are Brazil nuts, tuna, halibut, snapper, cod, shrimp, clams, oysters, sunflower seeds, whole grains, whole-wheat bread, and shitake and button mushrooms.

According to the World Health Organization (WHO), the recommended daily intake of selenium is 70 to 350 micrograms per day. Consuming too much of it (around 40 times of the recommended) is considered toxic.

2. **Iron** – This is the first of three trace metals that are considered as essential nutrients for thyroid health. All of the body's cells need iron to carry oxygen to its different parts, and also to store oxygen in the muscles. When it comes to the thyroid gland, iron helps in the production of thyroid hormones as well.

Iron-deficiency anemia, or not having enough iron in the blood, affects the efficacy of iodine in the body's systems. This reduces the performance of the thyroid. Iodine and iron work together to provide a steady balance in synthesizing thyroid hormones. Other effects of a lack of iron in the body are dizziness, fatigue, heart palpitations, irritability, cramping, hand numbness, diarrhea, loss of sex drive, and loss of appetite.

Foods that have high amounts of iron are seafood, poultry, red meat, dried fruit, peanuts, cashew nuts, almonds, lentils, white beans, and dark green leafy vegetables such as spinach, lettuce, cabbage, collard greens, mustard greens, and turnip greens.

The recommended daily allowance for iron varies from 7 to 27 milligrams a day, depending on age. Pregnant or breastfeeding mothers will also have a different requirement for iron intake.

3. **Zinc** – your thyroid also needs this trace metal to function properly. Zinc helps the hypothalamus, which is the part of the brain that connects the nervous system to the endocrine system, to produce Thyrotropin-Releasing Hormone or TRH. TRH triggers the pituitary gland's production of TSH (Thyroid-Stimulating Hormone). This in turn helps the thyroid to release its T_3 and T_4 hormones.

   When there is insufficient zinc in the body, there is also not enough TRH. The thyroid becomes slow and is put under stress, which causes hypothyroidism. However, when there is too much zinc in the body, the thyroid becomes too active, causing hyperthyroidism. The key is to only consume the right amount of zinc in your diet.

   Zinc is commonly found in oysters, portabella and shitake mushrooms, lean pork, lean poultry, beef, lamb, spinach, beans, pumpkin seeds, squash seeds, cashew nuts, and dark chocolate and cocoa.

   The recommended daily consumption is 3 to 40 milligrams per day. This recommended value could vary depending on age and whether a woman is pregnant or breastfeeding.

4. **Copper** – lastly, the third trace metal that the thyroid needs besides iron and zinc is copper. The relationship of copper with the thyroid gland is associated with zinc. This is because as an individual consumes more zinc in their diet, the copper levels in the body are reduced. This, of course, is not good. Copper provides many health benefits such as balancing the body's estrogen and progesterone levels, and regulating calcium in the vascular system to promote nutrient absorption.

On its own, copper is also good for the thyroid as it keeps the body from accumulating excess T_4 hormones in the bloodstream. It also keeps the thyroid healthy by controlling the release of thyroid hormones.

Common sources of copper are squid, octopus, crabs, lobsters, shrimps, oysters, shitake mushroom, chickpeas, kidney beans, sesame seeds, kale, avocadoes, and prunes and other dried fruits such as figs, apricots, and peaches.

It is recommended that about 340 to 1,000 micrograms of copper be consumed by the average individual per day. More than that is considered toxic.

5. **Vitamins A, C, and E** – these are antioxidant vitamins that help alleviate oxidative stress which can fatally affect the thyroid. Oxidative stress is perhaps the main reason for the development of many types of cancers, including thyroid cancer, and is also the main cause of Graves' disease, which is the most common type of hyperthyroidism. Antioxidants fight oxidation and the release of free radicals in the body.

Foods that contain vitamin A are spinach, kale, asparagus, lettuce, carrots, winter squash, sweet potatoes, and animal liver. Some vitamin C-rich foods are citrus fruits, tomatoes, papaya, strawberries, kiwi, guava, chili peppers, red bell peppers, green bell peppers, and kale. For vitamin E, the foods recommended are dark leafy vegetables, asparagus, beans, animal liver, almonds, peanuts, and sunflower seeds.

Recommended daily allowances for each are: vitamin A – 600 micrograms per day; vitamin C – 75 milligrams per day; and vitamin E – 10 milligrams per day.

6. **B vitamins** – the eight B vitamins are thiamin, riboflavin, niacin, pantothenic acid, pyridoxine, biotin, folate, and cobalamin. They are marked by the symbols B_1, B_2, B_3, B_5, B_6, B_7, B_9, and B_{12} respectively. They play a great role when it comes to proper cell metabolism. For the thyroid, B vitamins assist in the production of healthy and sufficient thyroid hormones, particularly T_4.

Foods that are high in B vitamins are:

- thiamin – dark green leafy vegetables, whole grain cereals

- riboflavin – milk, yogurt, cheese

- niacin – eggs, chicken, turkey, salmon, tuna, legumes, peanuts

- pantothenic acid and biotin – animal liver, egg yolks, salmon, avocado

- pyridoxine – seafood, poultry, dark green leafy vegetables, bananas, potatoes

- folate – grains, rice, spinach, turnip greens, fresh fruits and vegetables

- cobalamin – soy products, clams, mussels, crabs, beef

The recommended daily values for each B vitamin are:

- thiamin – 1.4 milligrams per day

- riboflavin – 1.2 milligrams per day

- niacin – 18 milligrams per day

- pantothenic acid – 6 milligrams per day

- pyridoxine – 2 milligrams per day

- biotin – 30 micrograms per day

- folate – 400 micrograms per day

- cobalamin – 6 micrograms per day

7. **Omega 3 fatty acids** – although there are still no official reports, medical experts are currently looking closely at the possible ways in which this polyunsaturated fatty acid improves thyroid conditions.

Fatty acids are essential to health as they are the main part of cell membranes. They also help in promoting proper cell growth, controlling inflammation, and relieving autoimmune diseases, such as many types of thyroiditis. This means that if a person has a thyroid condition that is autoimmune in nature, and they don't consume enough omega 3 in their diet, then the thyroid may go haywire.

Since the body cannot create omega 3 fatty acids on its own, it has to be taken through the person's diet. The major source of this nutrient is fish oil and seafood.

There is no recommended daily dosage for omega 3 fatty acid, although supplements are advised by most doctors.

Chapter 5:
Tips on Planning a Thyroid-Friendly Diet

A thyroid-friendly diet is so much more important than a weight loss diet. It is something that is needed to improve thyroid disorders, manage their symptoms, and improve proper metabolism. Moreover, it is not just about knowing what and what not to eat, but also knowing *how* and *how much* to eat.

Weight Loss and Gain

It is important to note that weight loss and weight gain are the common symptoms of hyperthyroidism and hypothyroidism, and not their causes. You don't get thyroid disorders from losing or gaining weight. When you have fewer thyroid hormones, your body burns lesser calories, which promotes weight gain. In contrast, excessive thyroid hormones tend to accelerate the metabolism, which makes you lose weight. It is important to consider these factors when planning your own diet.

The right diet for people with different thyroid disorders consists mostly of the same types of foods, only with different amounts or servings depending if one has excessive thyroid hormones (hyperthyroidism) or insufficient thyroid hormones (hypothyroidism).

In any case, however, a thyroid-friendly diet is really quite the same as that of what a normal person should be eating to stay healthy. It is always necessary to incorporate more fruits and vegetables in the diet, and have less sugar, caffeine, fatty foods, and processed foods.

Below are some tips on how to plan a thyroid-friendly diet:

1. Find the Right Substitutes

All types of diets basically want to cut down on sugar, caffeine, harmful fat, and processed foods. These same elements are especially detrimental for someone with a thyroid disorder. There are many ways to cut down on these damaging foods without torturing yourself. For example, if you have a really sweet tooth, then you can try a piece of fresh fruit or berries with whipped cream as a substitute for cake or other pastries. You can still have the same sweet flavor, but with more fresh food included in the serving.

2. Have as much Antioxidants as possible

If you are managing an autoimmune form of thyroid disorder, like Hashimoto's disease, you will need more antioxidants in your diet. Choose foods that are rich in vitamins A, C, and E, as these are great antioxidant vitamins, as mentioned in the previous chapter.

Dark green leafy vegetables (spinach, kale, arugula, lettuce, collards, and other greens), citrus fruits (oranges, grapefruit, lemon, lime, tangerine, and pomelo), and nuts and beans, should be the major components of your food intake. As mentioned in the previous chapter, antioxidants relieve oxidative stress that causes autoimmune thyroid conditions.

3. Organic is Better

As much as possible, it is better to eat organic food. For one, it contains lower amounts of chemicals, like insecticides, herbicides, and other forms of pesticides, that can further damage the thyroid. One of the major goals of a thyroid-friendly diet is to eliminate as much stress as possible from the thyroid gland, and organic foods are the best way to do this!

4. Keep Blood Sugar in Check

Erratic blood sugar fluctuations have a negative effect on the thyroid's physical properties. High blood sugar causes inflammation and swelling to the thyroid gland if not properly regulated. It is better to have six small meals of 300 calories in a day than have 3 large portions of 600 calories, for example. This is ideal, except for meals after strenuous workouts or activities, in which you need more carbohydrates to recover and compensate for the energy you have just burned.

5. Make Your Body More Alkaline

Cells function better in an alkaline environment rather than in an acidic one. On the other hand, an acidic system puts a lot of unnecessary stress on the body, leading to a slower metabolism and many deficiencies, including that of thyroid hormones. Too much alkalinity, however, is also not advised as the body may experience catabolism, where tissues and cells break down rapidly because of chemical stress. The ideal pH level of the body should be in between 6.5 to 7.5.

To have a more alkaline system, you simply have to include more fresh fruits and vegetables in your meals. Alkaline-inducing foods are those rich in calcium, zinc, potassium, and magnesium, such as carrots, eggplants, celery, cucumber, tomatoes, watercress, wheat grass, radishes, onions, kale, spinach, dandelions, rutabaga, sweet potatoes, and seaweeds.

Have smaller amounts of meat and dairy products because these protein-rich foods typically promote an acidic environment. However, eliminating protein completely from your diet will also have adverse effects on the thyroid, so it is important to find the right balance.

6. Consume Enough Protein

Speaking of protein, according to medical research, for each kilogram of body weight, an average person has to consume at least 800 milligrams of protein per day. However, this figure is not applicable for people who experience high stress levels. That is why 1.2 grams of protein per day is the most ideal for those who have thyroid conditions.

For best results, try to consume protein only from healthy sources such as fish, poultry, eggs, legumes, nuts, and organic dairy products.

7. Keep Yourself Hydrated

Water is the best friend of someone with a thyroid disorder. Not only does plain water support the optimal health of the thyroid gland, but it is also a great way to feel fuller whenever you get unhealthy food cravings. Water is also very good for preventing constipation, which is a common symptom of thyroid disorders. If you have to consume a beverage, your first choice should always be water.

8. Find the Right Balance

While there are foods that inhibit thyroid performance, such as cruciferous vegetables and soy products, it is important to keep in mind that they should not be completely taken away from a balanced diet. Consume them in moderation, and be sure to have enough thyroid-friendly foods in your diet to counter the negative effects.

Conclusion

Thank you again for downloading this book!

I hope this book was able to help you learn more about thyroid disorders!

The next step is to put this information to use, and begin improving your thyroid disorder with a change in diet!

Finally, if you enjoyed this book, please take the time to share your thoughts and post a review on Amazon. It'd be greatly appreciated!

Thank you and good luck!

www.ingramcontent.com/pod-product-compliance
Lightning Source LLC
Chambersburg PA
CBHW062345300326
41947CB00012B/1306